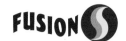

GET OUTDOORS

Go Camping!

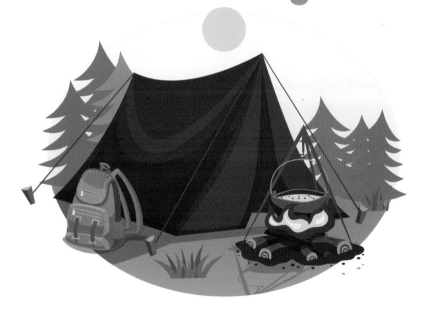

by Meghan Gottschall

BEARPORT
PUBLISHING

Minneapolis, Minnesota

President: Jen Jenson
Director of Product Development: Spencer Brinker
Senior Editor: Allison Juda
Designer: Colin O'Dea

Library of Congress Cataloging-in-Publication Data

Names: Gottschall, Meghan, author.
Title: Go camping! / by Meghan Gottschall.
Description: Minneapolis, Minnesota : Bearport Publishing Company, [2022] |
Series: Get outdoors | Includes bibliographical references and index.
Identifiers: LCCN 2020057402 (print) | LCCN 2020057403 (ebook) | ISBN 9781647479671 (library binding) |
   ISBN 9781647479749 (paperback) | ISBN 9781647479817 (ebook)
Subjects: LCSH: Camping--Juvenile literature.
Classification: LCC GV191.7 .G68 2022 (print) | LCC GV191.7 (ebook) | DDC 796.54--dc23
LC record available at https://lccn.loc.gov/2020057402
LC ebook record available at https://lccn.loc.gov/2020057403

For more information, write to Bearport Publishing, 5357 Penn Avenue South, Minneapolis, MN 55419. Printed in the United States of America.

Image Credits

Cover, © Colorlife/Shutterstock, © Merggy/Shutterstock, © Greenlate/Shutterstock, © Viktoriya Bronska/Shutterstock; 1M, © Macrovector/Shutterstock; 5T, © oliveromg/Shutterstock; 6BL, © OpenClipart-Vectors/Pixabay; 7, © Dan Howard/Getty Images; 8BL, © gresei/Shutterstock; 10BR, © lzf/Getty Images; 11TR, © PeopleImages/Getty Images; 11BR, © kedrov/Shutterstock; 11TM, © Pinkyone/Shutterstock; 11M, © Pixfiction/Shutterstock; 11TL, © Magdalena Wielobob/Shutterstock; 13B, © MemoryCatcher/Pixabay; 13M, © Tunatura/Shutterstock; 13T, © FabricioMacedoPhotos/ Pixabay; 14BR, © lady-luck/Shutterstock; 15, © Isaac Murray/Getty Images; 16BL, © veronicabuffalo/Pixabay; 17T, © Skorzewiak/Shutterstock; 18M, © Jazzmanian/Wikimedia; 19B, © Trusova Evgeniya/Shutterstock; 20M, © ittipon/Shutterstock; 21BM, © DeawSS/Shutterstock; 21BR, © Hatchapong Palurtchaivong/Shutterstock; 22M, © Beautiful landscape/Shutterstock; 23, © anatoliy_gleb/Shutterstock; Backgrounds: © Clker-Free-Vector-Images/Pixabay, © Merggy/Shutterstock; pattern, © Shirstok/Shutterstock; Design elements: © aliaksei kruhlenia/Shutterstock, © Janjf93/Pixabay, © NotionPic/Shutterstock, © JungleOutThere/ Shutterstock, © Kaliene/Pixabay, © Colorlife/Shutterstock, © Sudowoodo/Shutterstock

CONTENTS

CAMPING ADVENTURE

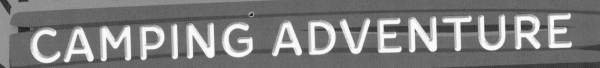

Hi, I'm Rory Raccoon, and I love to GET OUTDOORS!

Grab your tent and get ready to cozy up by the campfire. We're going camping!

There are so many things to do when you camp. Go **hiking** and look for wild animals. Try fishing in a river or lake.

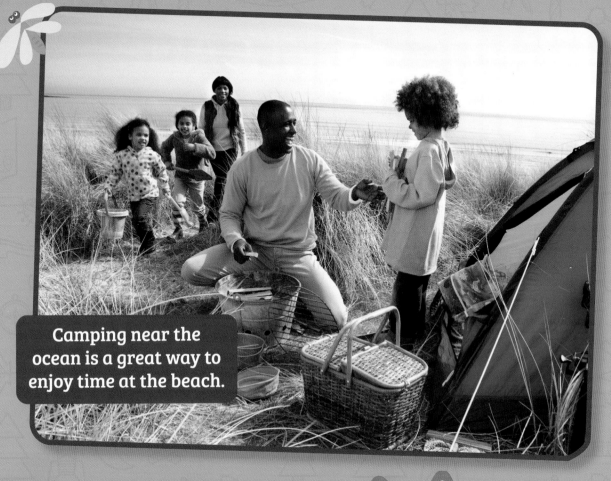

Camping near the ocean is a great way to enjoy time at the beach.

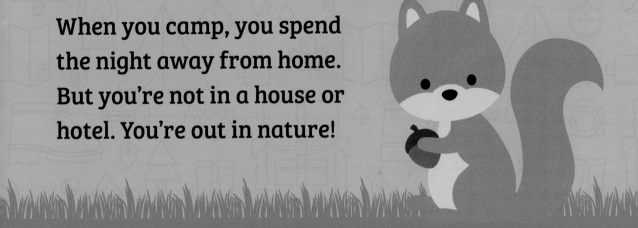

When you camp, you spend the night away from home. But you're not in a house or hotel. You're out in nature!

WHERE TO CAMP

Where will you go on your camping trip? You may want to stay at a **campground**. This is an area set up for people who are camping. There are campgrounds in **state parks** and **national parks**.

The first campground was opened in 1861.

Many campgrounds have bathrooms and showers. They might also have picnic tables.

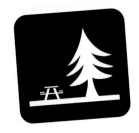

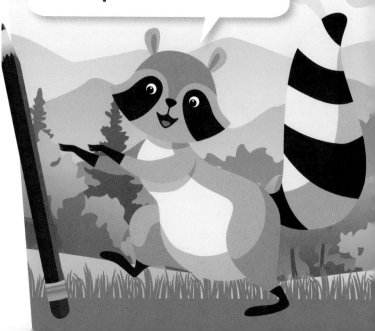

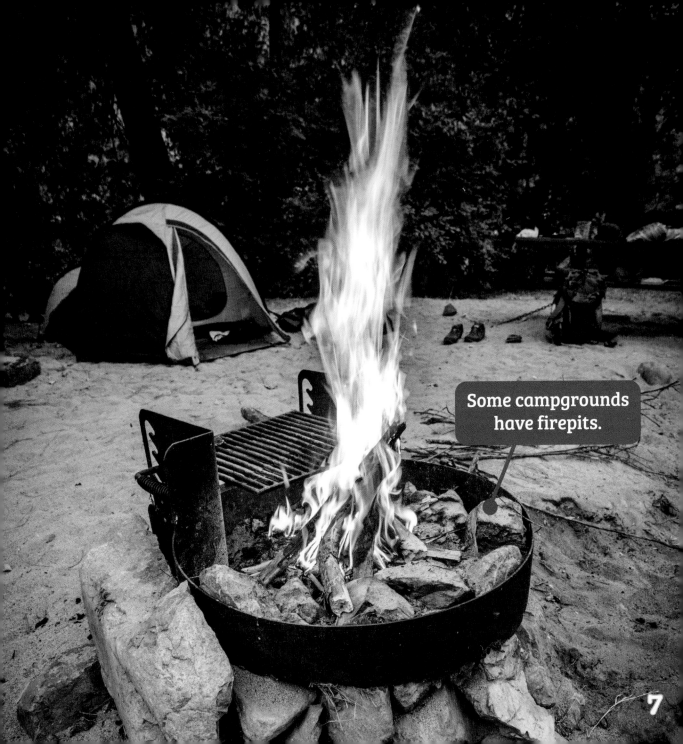

Some campgrounds have firepits.

GATHER YOUR GEAR

Before you begin your **adventure**, you'll need to pack. What should you bring? Grab a sleeping bag. It will keep you warm during cold nights. You can bring a pad to go under your sleeping bag. What other gear will you need to have a fun and safe camping trip?

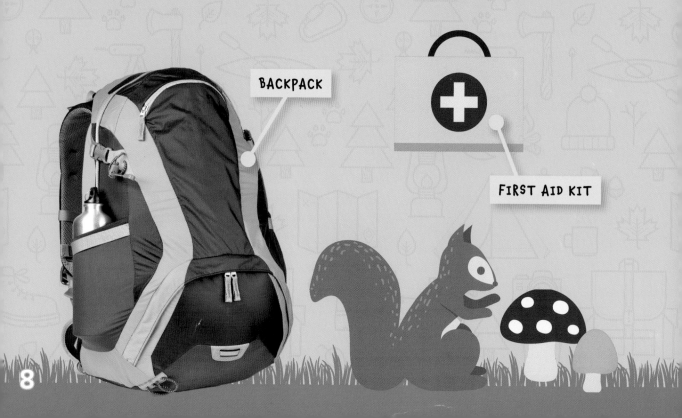

BACKPACK

FIRST AID KIT

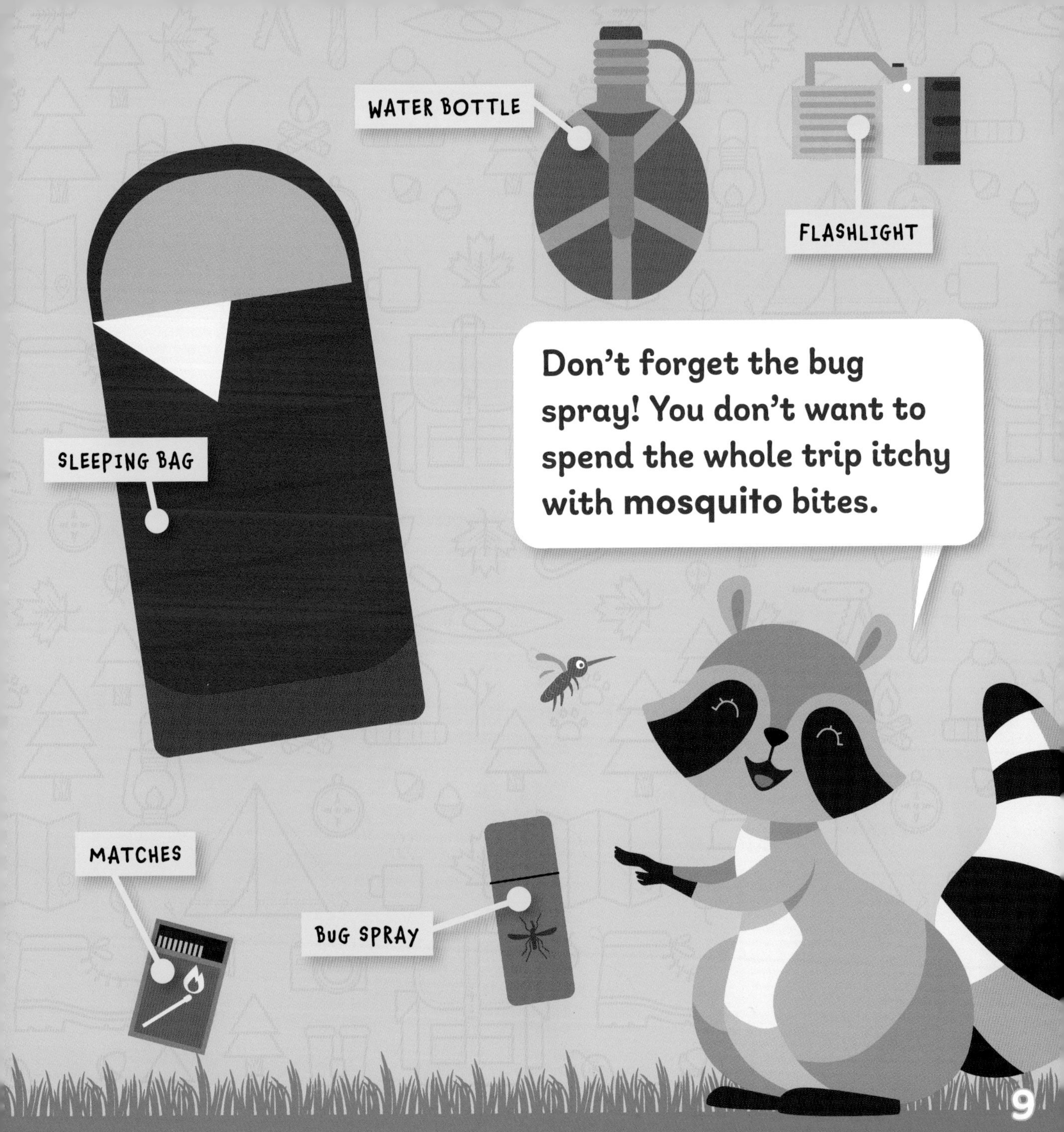
WATER BOTTLE
FLASHLIGHT
SLEEPING BAG
Don't forget the bug spray! You don't want to spend the whole trip itchy with mosquito bites.
MATCHES
BUG SPRAY

WHAT TO WEAR

What clothes should you bring? Leave your fancy clothes at home. Camping clothes should be easy to move in. You need to be ready for sun, rain, and maybe snow!

Hiking boots **protect** your feet from rocks. Long-sleeve shirts and long pants can stop bug bites.

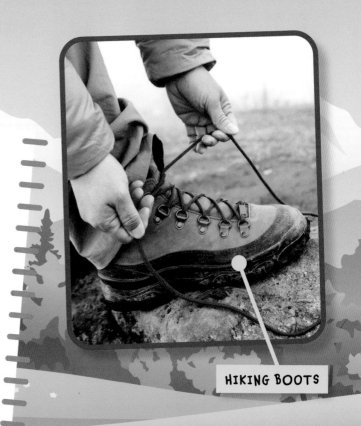

HIKING BOOTS

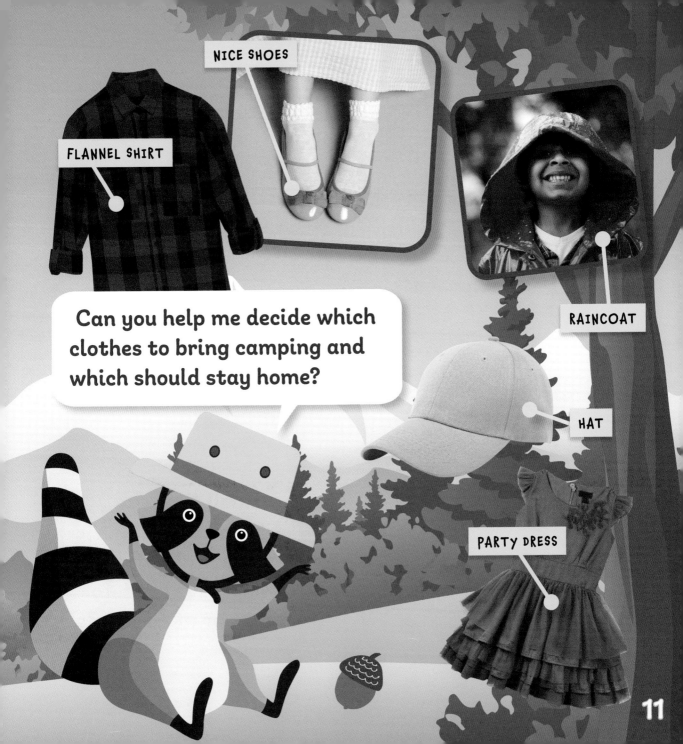

NICE SHOES

FLANNEL SHIRT

RAINCOAT

Can you help me decide which clothes to bring camping and which should stay home?

HAT

PARTY DRESS

11

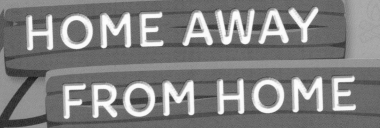

HOME AWAY FROM HOME

You've got your sleeping bag and clothes. But don't forget the most important part. You'll need your home away from home! Will you camp in a tent? Maybe you'll stay in an RV or pop-up camper.

A small tent can fit just one person inside. But some tents have room for eight or more people!

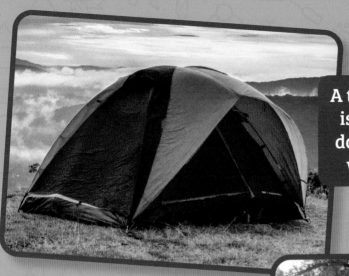

A tent is made of **fabric** that is held up by poles. It folds down to fit into a small bag when it's not being used.

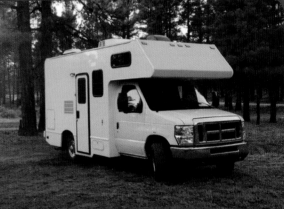

RVs are homes on wheels. They can have beds, small kitchens, and even bathrooms. Many campgrounds have places to park RVs.

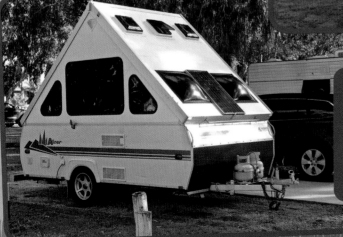

Pop-up campers are pulled by cars or trucks. They fold down so that they can be moved around. Then, you can open them up at the campsite.

SET UP CAMP

Let's camp in a tent! First, find some flat ground.
Then, clear away rocks, sticks, and pine cones.
Put down a **tarp** to keep the bottom of your tent
dry. Now you're ready to set up the tent!

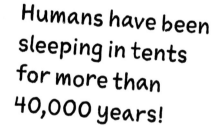

Humans have been
sleeping in tents
for more than
40,000 years!

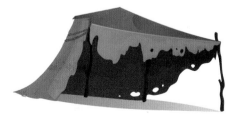

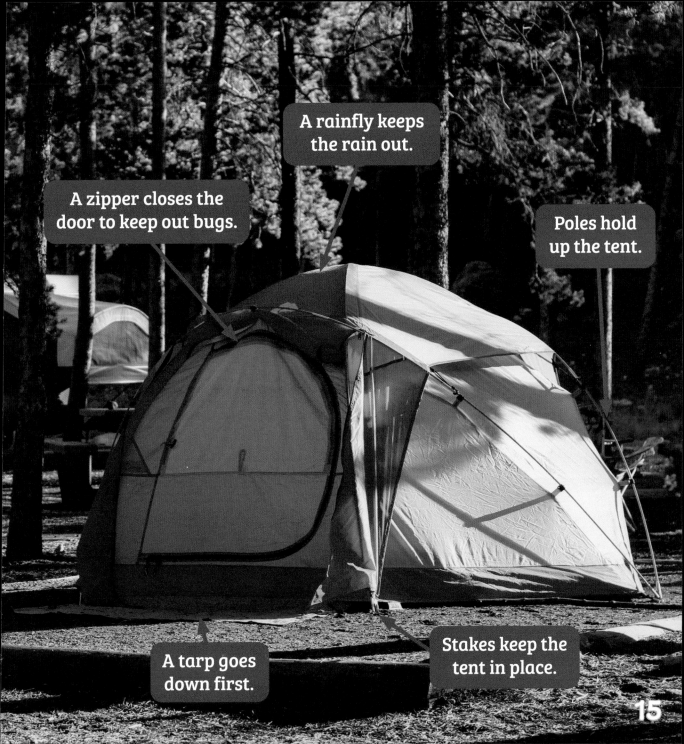

TIME TO EAT

What should you bring to eat when you're camping? Many kinds of food don't need to be cooked at all. Fruit, trail mix, and sandwiches are all good camping foods. To cook hot meals, you can use a camp stove.

Camp stoves don't need to be plugged in to work. They use **fuel**.

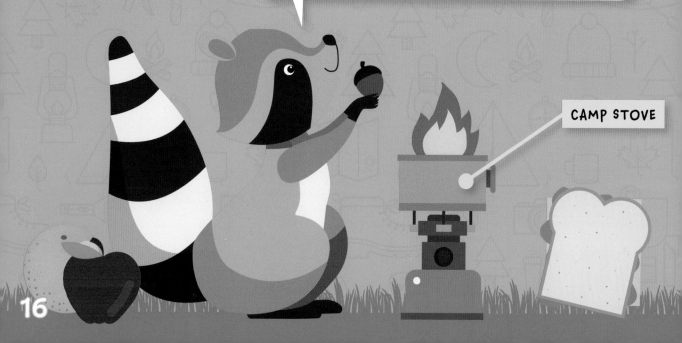

CAMP STOVE

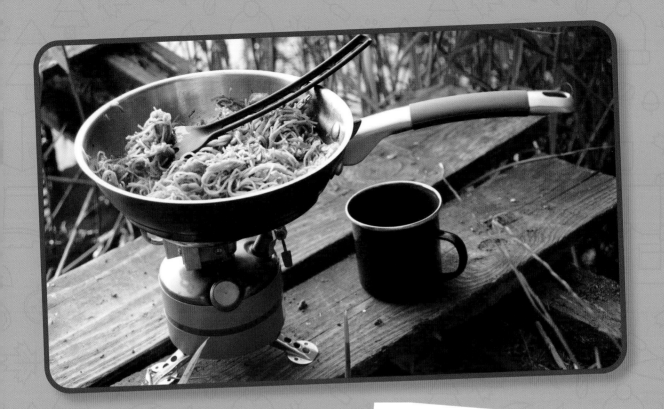

Camp stoves are small and don't hold very much fuel. You should choose food that is fast and easy to cook, such as pasta, canned soup, or oatmeal.

Don't leave any food outside when you're done. You don't want hungry bears or other animals to join you!

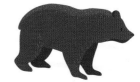

17

A COZY FIRE

You can also cook over a campfire. Hot dogs on a stick, anyone? To build a fire, find small sticks and put them in a pile. Then, add bigger pieces of wood. Ask an adult to light the fire.

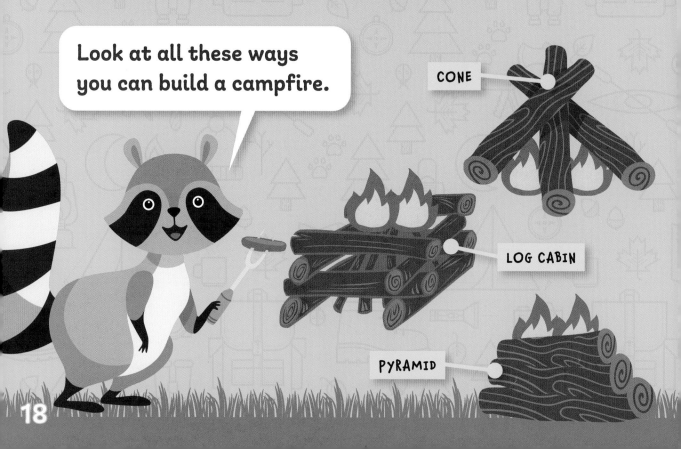

Look at all these ways you can build a campfire.

CONE

LOG CABIN

PYRAMID

When it's time for bed, make sure the fire is out all the way. First, put water on it. Then, cover it with dirt.

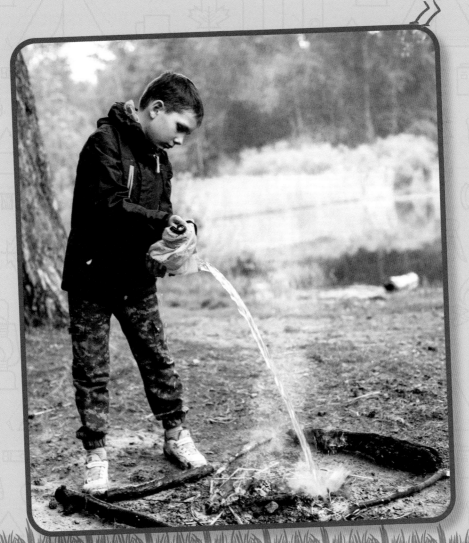

CLEANING UP

Good morning! Did you sleep well? Before you go home, there's one more thing to do. It's time to clean up.

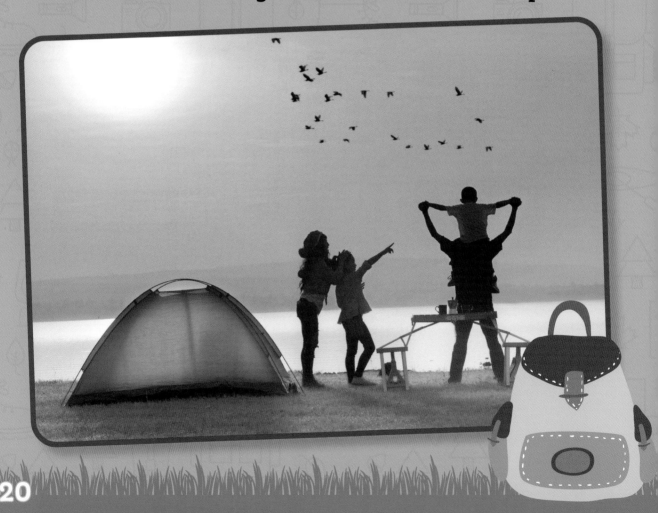

Picking up garbage keeps animals safe. It makes the area clean for other campers, too. Follow the rule called carry in, carry out. This means that anything you bring camping (carry in) should leave with you (carry out) or be thrown away correctly.

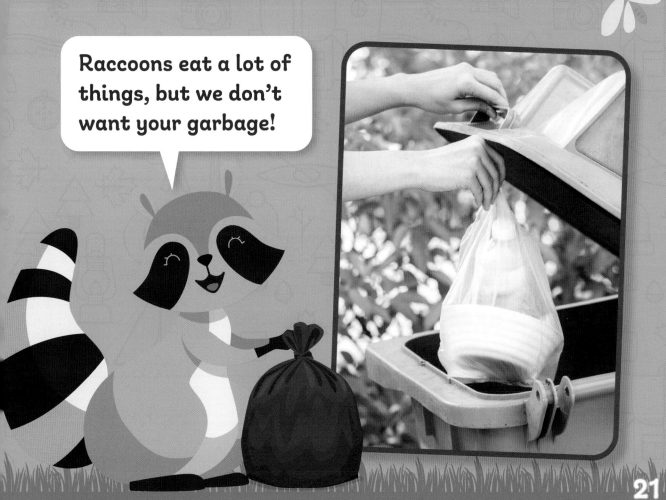

Raccoons eat a lot of things, but we don't want your garbage!

FUN FOR ALL

The next time you need a break, plan a camping trip! Setting up a tent, sitting around a campfire, and sleeping under the stars is so fun. Camping is a great way to spend time outdoors with family and friends.

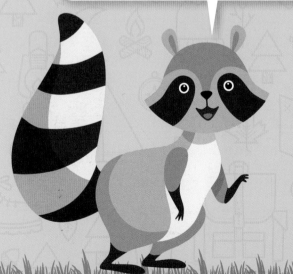

I can't wait to see you again the next time we GET OUTDOORS!

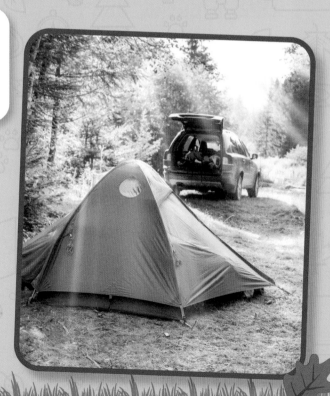

22

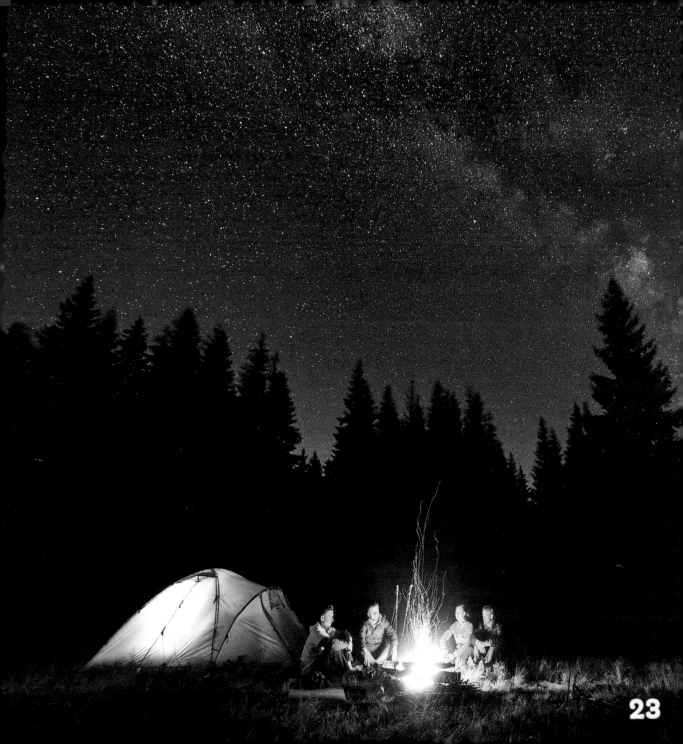

GLOSSARY

adventure an exciting experience

campground a place used for camping

fabric cloth, or other material made from woven fibers

fuel material, such as gas, that is burned to create heat

hiking walking long distances for fun or exercise

mosquito a small flying insect that bites people and animals

national parks areas of land set aside by the U.S. government to protect the animals and plants that live there

protect to keep safe

state parks areas of land set aside by state governments to protect the animals and plants that live there

tarp a heavy, waterproof piece of fabric

INDEX